Female Anesthesiologist

Author : Hala Mostafa Goma ,MD, professor of Anesthesia ,Cairo University

Table Of contents

Introduction

Women in Egypt are the first in invading the medical field in the Arab world. They started at the end of the 21 century. At first they were in nursing field, after that they entered the medical field as pediatric, obstetric fields. Anesthesia field was a difficult field for the Arab women.1966 the first female anesthesiologist was in the medical field in Egypt. Till now Female anesthesiologists are facing many problems, and fighting for long time to be confident and to convince their community to be equal in anesthesia as male anesthesiologists. In this book I tried to summary the problems and the challenges that face the female anesthesiologist.

Author Recommendations:

Support female anesthesiologist especially in developing countries. Starting to narrow the family gap,

Maternity leave adjustment for:

1. Keeping skills and experience by extended courses of training for female anesthesiologist with children.
2. Financial support for female anesthesiologist, maintain children welfare as much as time spent with them.
3. The community and country development may use the double benefit from continuous support of working women, from her work, and from normal physical and emotional children.
4. Continuous medical super vision against hazards of infection and radiation ,with special attention during pregnancy.
5. Community support motivates working women to get achievement in both work and children.

Factors affecting women in being anesthesiologist:

1-Economic factors:

Medical studying is expensive, and need special sponsoring of colleges. in Arabs countries the family is responsible about the financial support. Many families cannot afford. Training of anesthesiologist needs to be also sponsored. The governmental support plays a role in training programs.

2-social factors:

The distant between colleges and students place of residence may play important role, with the presence of adequate safety for transportation.

3-Familial factors:

Family support is needed because the prolonged years of studying delayed age of marriage which considered important in Arab countries.

4-continous education:

The academic field of anesthesia needs continued financial support, and ,and adequate source of knowledge.

5-cultural factors:

Male anesthesiologists may be defective in proper cooperation with their female colleges; it may be due to the deeply inserted ideas about sex discrimination between males and females.

Private work may be restricted on male anesthesiologist by male surgeons.

The patients and their families may be not trust female anesthesiologist.

Infection and the female anesthesiologist:

i.   Operating room infection

ii.   Other hospital infection due contact with patients preoperatively or in ICU

Operating room infection:

Infection due to blood borne pathogens:

Risk of blood born infection

- Number of exposures to infected blood or body fluids.

- Prevalence of patients carrying the pathogen within an anaesthetist's practice.

- Infectivity of a particular pathogen

Blood born transmitted diseases

- Human immunodeficiency virus (HIV)
- Hepatitis B, and C.
- Prevention
- Effective clothing.
- Eye ware.
- Source of infection.

Transmission may also occur after exposure to body fluids other than blood, including amniotic fluid, cerebrospinal fluid, pericardial fluid, pleural fluid, synovial fluid, unfixed tissues and organs, exudative fluid from burns or skin lesions, vaginal secretions and semen

Method of infection:

Inoculation of pathogens by sharp ,needle, vascular ,CVP, spinal, or through wounded exposed hands

Hepatitis C infection:

- Hepatitis C contaminated occupational exposure has been estimated at 2%.
- Chronic hepatitis develops in 85% of hepatitis C infections .
- 20% progressing to cirrhosis and 3% to hepatocellular carcinoma.
- A chronic carrier state may also develop.
- No vaccine exists but some institutions offer immune serum globulin as post-exposure prophylaxis.

Acute phase:

The period immediately following infection is called the 'acute phase'. This lasts about six months.

chronic phase.

If the immune system does not manage to clear the virus in this time, the disease is considered to have moved into a long-term infection.

- Because of the damage it can cause to the liver, HCV is classified as a liver disease. But HCV can also affect some of the body's other systems, causing symptoms, illnesses and complications other than those associated with the liver.

- Until recently these other symptoms have often been seen as unconnected or unrelated. This has meant that they have been given less medical attention and, as a result, are less well researched and understood.
- The effects of hepatitis C on the liver are measured by the way the liver changes as scarring develops.
- This progression begins with the initial inflammation of the liver caused by the virus hijacking its cells. It then starts to infect and kill off the liver cells, before the gradual scarring (fibrosis) and then the hardening of the liver tissue (cirrhosis) occurs.
- Although it acts to source the spread of disease, it also enhances the process of scarring.
- Cirrhosis scars and alters the actual structure of the liver.
- Over time this will seriously undermine the liver's ability to function properly.
- Cirrhosis is classified as being either 'compensated' or 'decompensated '

Manifestations of decompensated cirrhosis:

- Portal Hypertension - when blood cannot properly flow through the liver and pressure rises in the portal vein leading into the liver.
- Variceal Bleeding - when the portal hypertension forces blood to re-route through veins that are too small and consequently burst, often in the esophagus (between the throat and the stomach), causing potentially life-threatening internal bleeding.
- Edema - when the liver stops producing enough albumins. This regulates the amount of fluid in cells. This fluid then builds up, typically in the stomach, and is known as ascites.
- Hepatic Encephalopathy - when the liver stops properly filtering poisons and toxins. These then build up in the brain leading to serious mental confusion and sometimes coma.

The risk of acquiring HIV after an occupational exposure to HIV-infected blood:

- The risk is low.
- Epidemiological studies have indicated that the risk for HIV transmission after percutaneous exposure to HIV-infected blood in health care settings is 0.3%.
- After a mucocutaneous exposure, the risk is 0.03% .
- If intact skin is exposed to HIV-infected blood there is no risk of HIV transmission.
- Several factors have been identified as types of exposure with significant potential to transmit HIV occupational exposure. The minimum dose of contaminated blood needed to infect a human after an occupational exposure is unknown

Effects of parntral infection and female anesthetist:

1. **Draw back and physical fitness.**
2. **Relation with her partner.** The risk of sexual transmission is small - maximum of 5%, but possibly much less. There is insufficient evidence firmly to recommend barrier contraception in stable monogamous relationships but is strongly advised for HCV-infected patients with multiple sexual partners.
3. **Pregnancy and parenteral infection:**

   - Discuss childbearing intentions with all women of childbearing age on an ongoing basis throughout the course of their care.
   - Provide information about effective and appropriate contraceptive methods to reduce the likelihood of unintended pregnancy.
   - During preconception counseling, include information on safer sexual practices and elimination of alcohol, illicit drugs, and smoking
   - All HIV-infected women contemplating pregnancy should be receiving combination antiretroviral therapy (cART) and have plasma
   - Viral load below the limit of detection prior to conception.
   - When selecting or evaluating cART for HIV-infected women of childbearing age, consider a regimen's effectiveness, a woman's
   - Hepatitis B status, teratogenic potential of the drugs in the cART regimen, and possible adverse outcomes for the mother and fetus.

- HIV infection does not preclude the use of any contraceptive method. However, drug-drug interactions between hormonal
- Contraceptives and cART should be taken into account.
- Recommendations for Use of Antiretroviral Drugs during Pregnancy
- Potential teratogenic effects and other short- and long-term adverse effects on fetuses or newborns
- including preterm birth, mutagenicity, and carcinogenicity,
- Experience with use in pregnancy,
- Potential drug interactions with other medications,
- Results of genotypic resistance testing and prior antiretroviral exposure,
- Pharmacokinetic (PK) changes in pregnancy and degree of placental transfer,
- Potential adverse maternal drug effects that may be exacerbated during pregnancy,
- Comorbidities,
- Ability of patient to adhere to regimen, and
- Convenience.

4- Increase risk of preterm labour and cesarean section.

5- Mother to baby (before or during birth); transmission rate from mother to child is about 6%.[4] However, this is increased to around 14-17% when there is co-infection with HIV.

6- Hepatitis c patients have increased risk of the following diseases

- o Diabetes.
- o Sjögren's syndrome.
- o Essential mixed cryoglobulinaemia.
- o Polyarteritis nodosa.
- o Autoimmune hepatitis.
- o Thyroiditis.
- o Membranous glomerulonephritis.
- o Porphyria cutanea tarda.
- o Lichen planus.
- o Immune thrombocytopenia.

- All cases of antiretroviral (ARV) drug exposure during pregnancy should be reported to the Antiretroviral Pregnancy Registry http://www.APRegistry.com)
- Non-pregnant women of childbearing potential should undergo pregnancy testing before initiation of efavirenz and receive counseling about the potential risk to the fetus and desirability of avoiding pregnancy while on efavirenz-containing regimens (AIII).
- Alternate ARV regimens that do not include efavirenz should be considered in women who are planning to become pregnant or are sexually active and not using effective contraception, assuming these alternative regimens are not thought to compromise a Woman's health (BIII).
- Efavirenz can be continued in women receiving an efavirenz-based regimen who present for antenatal care in the first trimester.

- Because the risk of neural tube defects is restricted to the first 5 to 6 weeks of pregnancy. Pregnancy is rarely recognized before 5 to
- 6 weeks, and unnecessary changes in ARV drugs during pregnancy may be associated with loss of viral control and increased risk of
- Perinatal transmission. In such situations, fetal ultrasound is recommended at 18 to 20 weeks to assess anatomy.

MANAGEMENT OF OCCUPATIONAL EXPOSURE

Post exposure management is important to be started once exposure occurs, to limit the drawback effects on both doctor and prevents further dissemination of infection.

Exposure Reporting

- Prevention remains the best strategy for protecting HCWs from occupationally acquired infection.

- Anesthetists should have written protocols for rapid reporting, evaluation, counseling, treatment, and

- Follow-up of work-related exposures that may place a worker at risk of blood-borne pathogen infection.

- Established exposure control plans and comply with incident reporting requirements mandated by OSHA.

- Access to clinicians who can provide post exposure care should be available during all work hours, including nights and weekends.

- post exposure counseling personals should be familiar with evaluation and treatment protocols and the facility's procedures for obtaining drugs for PEP

- After any exposure, efforts should be made to identify and evaluate clinically and epidemiologically the source patient for evidence of HIV, HBV, and/or HCV infection.

- The source patient should be informed of the incident and consent should be obtained for HIV, HBV, and HCV testing.

- ZDV and other reverse transcriptase inhibitors may be important for PEP by preventing early viral dissemination.

Post exposure Chemoprophylaxis for HIV

First aid should be administered as quickly as possible.

- Puncture wounds and other cutaneous injury sites should be washed with soap and water,

- Exposed oral and nasal mucous membranes should be strongly washedwith water.

- Eyes should be washed with clean water, saline, or sterile irrigants.

- Antiseptics for wound care is not evidenced based reduce the risk of blood-borne pathogen transmission, their use is not contraindicated. Avoid use of bleach or other caustic agents that cause local tissue trauma.

Post exposure Prophylaxis for HBV:

- Immunization of anesthetists with hepatitis B vaccine and hepatitis B IG .

- Management of HCWs after percutaneous (e.g., needlestick, laceration, or bite) or mucosal (e.g., mucous membrane or ocular) exposure to potentially infectious body fluids.

- HBsAg status of the source of exposure.

- Hepatitis B vaccination and vaccine response status of the exposed anesthetists.

Transmission of HCV from Infected **anesthetists** to Patients

- There are no reported cases of HCV transmission from infected surgeons or dentists to patients in the United States.

- Inform health department.

- Post-exposure prophylaxis has been shown to be maximally effective if taken within an hour after an exposure, but benefit may remain if commenced up to 2 weeks after exposure.

Hepatitis B infection:

- Hepatitis B is highly infectious and the risk of transmission after occupational exposure is higher than for HIV.
- The incidence of seroconversion from a high infectivity carrier (e antigen positive) to a non-immune health care worker is up to 40% after exposure by percutaneous inoculation, depending on the magnitude of contact with the blood.
- An effective vaccine exists to prevent the transmission of hepatitis B and all anesthetists should ensure that they are up to date with their immunization schedule.
- A blood test is necessary to confirm immunity as the non-responder rate is 5–10% and boosters are required every 5 yr.

- Anesthetists in whom no antibodies are present and who suspect exposure to hepatitis B should be immunized passively with hepatitis B immunoglobulin and receive a series of three injections of hepatitis B vaccine.
- Prior vaccination with seroconversion eliminates the need for immunoglobulin.

Tuberculosis and female anesthesiologist:

- In developing countries, prevalence of TB parallels its prevalence in the general population and kills more women of reproductive age than all the combined causes of maternal mortality.
- Tuberculosis spreads by small (1–5 μm) droplets released from an infected person.

Factors concerned in the transmission of the bacillus to an anesthetist

- Bronchoscopy, laryngoscopy, tracheal intubation, suctioning of the airways and mechanical ventilation.
- Probability of transmission is also related to the concentration of infectious droplets and
- Duration and repetition of the exposure.

Strategies to prevent disease transmission include:

- education to raise awareness;
- the use of appropriate protective clothing and personal respirators;
- limiting the number of personnel in contact with the patient

- Possible delaying surgery until a patient is non-infectious.
- A tuberculin test Screen test for Anesthetists who have experienced a high risk exposure.
- Indicated undertake 6–12 months of chemoprophylaxis.

Early diagnosis of TB

- increased respiratory rate fatigue
- Cough (74%),
- Weight loss (41%), fever (30%).
- Malaise and fatigue (30%) was found to be a common presenting manifestation of TB with pregnancy
- It can be easily seen that except weight loss (which to some extent can be compensated by weight gain during pregnancy)

TB test

TB test also has its higher pitfalls and fallacies when used during pregnancy; early studies showed false-negative skin tests

BCG vaccination

- o Areas of the world where TB is common and BCG vaccination is universal, tuberculin test more often confuses than contributes to the diagnosis.
- o important diagnostic tools is chest X-ray and this is usually avoided during pregnancy.

Tuberculosis and female reproductive health

- Female reproductive system is very vulnerable to this infection and clinical presentation of this disease in female reproductive tract is variable in character
- A large majority of patients could be completely silent.
- This disease is an important cause of infertility, menstrual irregularity, pregnancy loss, and in association with pregnancy, morbidity to both the mother and child increases.
- Some of the effects of TB infection on female genital tract could be remote in nature due to systemic infection.
- Medicines used to treat TB infection can also have adverse effects on contraception and other areas of female reproductive health.
- HIV confection and multidrug-resistant tuberculosis (MDR-TB) and increased.
- Disordered menstruation.
- The pregnancy outcome in a subset of patients.
- TB if self-mimicking pregnancy or certain pregnancy related complications.
- Chances of causing TB in the neonate.
- Ability of the Antitubercular drugs to increase certain complications in pregnant woman.
- Antitubercular drug and its teratogenic potential.
- Recent increase in MDR-/XDR-TB.
- Infertility.

- Challenges of increased load of genital TB in females from the developing countries.

Disordered menstruation

- Weight loss and is associated with systemic inflammatory response and cachexia can cause amenorrhea.
- TB affects adrenal gland (used to be one of the common causes of Addison's disease in the past), pituitary gland and ovaries
- hypomenorrhea or amenorrhea has been described in a substantial number
- Hormonal changes which can affect menstruation have been observed in these patients
- anti-gonadotrophic effect of *M. tuberculosis* has been demonstrated in the studies
- Pulmonary TB patients have endometrial involvement.
- Rifampicin", has been shown to induce menstrual disturbances.
- Antitubercular therapy adds other dimensions to the cause of amenorrhea in this condition.
- Rifampicin-induced increased enzymatic catabolism of estrogens may affect Luteinizing Hormone surge, resulting in an ovulating cycle.
- Menorrhagia is uncommon; this can follow when TB causes tubo-ovarian mass or Following an ovulatory cycle.

pathological effects of TB mon female genital system

o Fallopian tube (92-100%), ovaries (10-30%), endometrium (50%), cervix (5%) and rarely vagina or vulva (<1%).

o Uterine synechiae is also an important cause of secondary amenorrhea associated with TB.

TB and pregnancy

- Pregnancy does not influence the course of pulmonary or extrapulmonary TB.

- But there are some reports of the aggravation of the condition during pregnancy.

- In advanced countries when TB is diagnosed early and treated, TB rarely influences the outcome of pregnancy.

- 90% of TB occurs and pregnant woman with TB often presents late to the Gynecologist for management.
- MDR-/XDR-TB increasingly involves pregnant woman

Maternal complication

Rates with both pulmonary and extrapulmonary TB are increased

a) Pregnancy associated hypertension (8.6%).

b) Respiratory failure (5.8%) .

c) Oligohydramnios (2.9%).

d) Relative risk of overall maternal complication was 3.1 and preterm labor was increased eightfold

e) Higher frequency of toxemia, abortion and intrapartum complications has also been reported

f) Fetal growth retardation was noted in several studies.

g) Overall incidence of perinatal mortality is high where TB has affected pregnancy.

h) pulmonary, meningeal and miliary TB

i) Active TB of spine can cause deformation of pelvis or obstructed labor. TB of spine can also cause paraplegia and may be associated with delayed progression of labor due to loss of Fergusson reflex. Vaginal delivery is not contraindicated in such cases, but spinal nursing in a patient with rapidly enlarging uterus can pose a challenge.

TB itself mimicking pregnancy and pregnancy associated complications:

Abdominal TB coupled with amenorrhea in females may mimic pregnancy superficially.

- sonography machines have reached the remote corners of many developing nations.
- Abdominal distension, pain, amenorrhea of abdominal TB with pregnancy
- Misdiagnosing abdominal TB with pregnancy.

Complications with associated pregnancy may mimic pregnancy complications, for example, increased urinary frequency with pyuria of renal TB may mimic urinary tract infection of pregnancy and repeated vomiting during pregnancy may be confused with hyperemesis gravidarum (HG).

TB in the neonate:

- The overall mortality for neonatal TB is high (38% in untreated and 22% in the treated.
- A fetus can get TB infection from the mother either through ingestion or aspiration of infected amniotic fluid
- Hematogenous from ulcers in the lower genital tract during delivery spread through umbilical vein to fetal liver via placental TB.
- True congenital TB seems to be rare, but infection after birth from the mother, particularly if mother has open cavitary TB and has been on anti-TB drug for less than 2 weeks.

Congenital criteria

1) Primary hepatic comple
2) Caseating granuloma by percutaneous liver biopsy at birth
3) the presence of maternal genital tract lesion due to TB
4) TB placentitis
5) The presence of tubercular infection in the neonate in the first week of life where postnatal transmission has been ruled out by proper investigation of contacts including the attendants.

ciinical picture of infected neonate

1. A neonate presenting with TB may present with respiratory distress,
2. fever, poor feeding, lethargy, irritability,
3. Abdominal distension, lymphadenopathy or hepatosplenomegaly.
4. Favorable response is not obtained with broad-spectrum antibiotics and investigations for other congenital infections are negative, then TB should be high on the list.
5. Chest radiography is abnormal in most of the patients and 50% of such patients have military TB.

Protection of the neonate from TB

- BCG vaccination is given at birth; it may take another 3-4 weeks before hypersensitivity to TB develops.
- Once TB is diagnosed, standard treatment with Antitubercular drugs may be initiated.

- INH prophylaxis (5 mg/kg) can be given to exposed neonates, and in developed countries, BCG vaccination may be given at 3 months of age if the child is still tuberculin negative.

Side effects of antitubercular drugs:

symptoms like gastric irritation, neuropathy (if given without vitamin B6),

Drug fever, thrombocytopenia,

Neuropsychiatric manifestations, optic neuropathy (Ethambutol)

Fulminant hepatitis.

Second-line drugs

- Treatment with first-line drugs during pregnancy is considered safe for both mother and the fetus.
- Deafness, convulsion, neuropsychiatric changes
- aminoglyocosides, poses a very high risk of fetal deafness
- Ethionamide, Proethionamide, and Cycloserine should not be used for pregnancy either because of lack of information or possible teratogenic effect
- Rifampicin and INH freely cross placenta and Rifampicin has been associated with 4.4% fetal malformation rate.
- Ethambutol is associated with 2.2% malformation rate

- All the first-line antitubercular drugs are compatible with breast feeding. .

MDR-/XDR-TB associated with pregnancy

Limited number of studies on MDR-/XDR-TB with pregnancy .

Infertility and sub fertility associated with TB of the genital tract:

- Incidence of infertility in genital TB varied from 10 to 85%.
- Genital TB invariably affects the fallopian tube, and in 50% of the cases of genital TB, endometrial is also involved.
- Genital TB not only causes tubal obstruction,
- impairs implantation due to endometrial involvement
- Ovulatory failure from ovarian involvement.
- Synechiae of the endometrium.
- Hysteroscopy and hysterosalpingography
  Successful pregnancy is extremely low in patients with genital TB even after complete treatment of TB.

- Repeated IVF failure if the disease is not diagnosed beforehand and treated.

Female anesthesiologists and, radiation:

Types of radiation:

    1) Ionizing radiation from X-rays, CT, MRI.

    2) Non-ionizing radiation from lasers.

- Exposure from lasers may occur through direct exposure or reflection. Resulting injuries include burns to the cornea and retina, destruction of the macula or optic nerve and cataract formation.
- Protective eyewear is designed to filter out radiation produced by specific lasers and should be worn at all times when lasers are in use.

Dose of exposure:

It is very small but repeated cumulative exposure may be hazardous.

The monthly cumulative dose of of the annual radiation exposure calculated to be below the dose limit of 15 mSv yr^{-1}.

Places for anesthesiologist exposure to radiation:

- Operating rooms of orthopedic operations, neurosurgical, urosurgical, and trauma theaters where direct exposure may occur.
- In diagnostic labs as in MRI, CT, Urological images, and ERCP, Gastroenterology diagnostic images.

Magnetic resonance imaging (MRI):

MRI intense magnetic field exposure hazards:

- **Acoustic noise**

  Acoustic noise is produced by the vibration of the switched gradient coils during MRI scanning.

  Hypoxia:

- Cryogens, usually liquid helium, are used to maintain the magnetic coils at superconducting temperature.

- Quenching is the rapid boil-off of the cryogen which may occur because of system failure, or if the magnetic field needs to be shut down rapidly. The resultant large volumes of gas should be safely vented to the outside atmosphere; however, if this is prevented, the rapid production of helium gas could result in a hypoxic atmosphere.

  projectile effect on ferromagnetic

  Intense magnetic fields can cause projectile effect on ferromagnetic.

  Movement or malfunction of the Implanted ferromagnetic items

  As aneurysm clips or pacemakers may with potentially fatal results **nausea or vertigo** from stimulation of the semicircular canals.

  Occupational Radiation Exposure Based on the National Dose Registry of Canada:

  1. elevated standardized incidence ratios for thyroid cancer and melanoma;

2. Elevated excess relative risks for rectum, leukemia, lung, all cancers combined, all except lung, and all except leukemia.

3. For males, cancers of the colon, pancreas, and testis also showed significantly elevated excess relative risks.

4. The thyroid standardized incidence ratios in this study are highly significant, but further investigation is needed to assess the possibility of association with occupational radiation exposure.

5. The standardized incidence ratio for melanoma was significantly elevated in males. Excess relative risks of cancer, Canadian National Dose Registry cohort, 1969–1988.

6. Colon, Rectum, Pancreas, Larynx Lung, Melanoma Prostate Testis, Bladder Non-Hodgkin's lymphoma Leukemia, Leukemia excluding chronic lymphatic leukemia Myeloid or monocytic leukemia Acute myeloid or monocytic leukemia.

First Analysis of Cancer Incidence and Occupational Radiation Exposure Based on the National Dose Registry of Canada

TABLE 5.

Standardized incidence ratios for females, Canadian National Dose Registry cohort, 1969–1988*

	No. of cases			90%
Cancer type	**Observed**	**Expected**	**SIR†**	**CI†**
Tongue and mouth	7	12.4	0.56	0.26, 1.06

Cancer type	No. of cases		SIR†	90% CI†
	Observed	Expected		
Salivary gland	7	7.1	0.98	0.46, 1.85
Pharynx	6	9.1	0.66	0.29, 1.29
Esophagus	7	5.1	1.36	0.64, 2.56
Stomach	21	28	0.75	0.50, 1.08
Colon	105	113	0.93	0.79, 1.10
Rectum	40	50.6	0.79	0.60, 1.03
Liver	7	5.2	1.33	0.63, 2.51
Gallbladder	4	8.9	0.45	0.15, 1.02
Pancreas	18	23.2	0.78	0.50, 1.15

Cancer type	No. of cases		SIR†	90% CI†
	Observed	Expected		
Nose	2	3	0.67	0.12, 2.11
Larynx	6	7.3	0.82	0.36, 1.62
Lung	92	116	0.79	0.66, 0.94
Bone	6	8.8	0.69	0.30, 1.35
Connective and soft tissue	20	17.4	1.15	0.76, 1.67
Melanoma	105	94.3	1.11	0.94, 1.31
Breast	544	584	0.93	0.87, 1.00
Uterus including cervix	193	271	0.71	0.63, 0.80
Ovary	105	98.4	1.07	0.90, 1.25

Cancer type	No. of cases		SIR†	90% CI†
	Observed	Expected		
Bladder	20	29.2	0.68	0.45, 1.00
Kidney	21	26.5	0.79	0.53, 1.14
Brain, nervous system	29	44.8	0.65	0.46, 0.88
Thyroid gland‡	94	66.1	1.42	1.19, 1.69
Non-Hodgkin's lymphoma	41	58.2	0.71	0.53, 0.91
Hodgkin's disease	36	37	0.97	0.72, 1.28
Multiple myeloma	6	11.1	0.54	0.24, 1.07
Leukemia	30	42.6	0.70	0.51, 0.96
Leukemia excluding chronic lymphatic leukemia	27	35.9	0.75	0.53, 1.04

Cancer type	No. of cases		SIR†	90% CI†
	Observed	Expected		
Myeloid or monocytic leukemia	21	25	0.84	0.56, 1.21
Acute myeloid or monocytic leukemia	12	15.5	0.77	0.45, 1.25
Other cancers	72	85.6	0.84	0.69, 1.02
All cancers	1,639	1,856	0.88	0.85, 0.92

Data are based on first diagnosis. Skin cancers other than melanoma are excluded from the analysis. Uranium miners are not included in the cohort.

† SIR, standardized incidence ratio; CI, confidence interval.

Significantly elevated SIR

W. N. Sont [1] ,J. M. Zielinski [2] , J. P. Ashmore [1] , H. Jiang [3] , D. Krewski [4] ,

M. E. Fair [5] ,P. R. Band [2] and E. G. Létourneau: **First Analysis of Cancer Incidence and Occupational Radiation Exposure Based on the National Dose Registry of Canada**   Oxford JournalsMedicine & Health American Journal of EpidemiologyVolume 153, Issue 4 **Pp. 309-318**

Protection of anesthesiologist against radiation:

1. Careful applications of time, distance, and shielding affect dose.
2. Suitable use includes collimating properly, optimizing beam-on time, minimizing distances between image intensifier and patient.
3. Ensuring adequate distance between patient and x-ray tube, and optimizing exposure rates for image quality and dose.
4. Dose limits typically regulate maximum whole-body dose.
5. Protective clothing worn by fluoroscopists reduces personnel risks.
6. Weighting factors can be useful to estimate effective dose equivalent.
7. Pregnant personnel have lower limits, which apply only with controlled declaration of pregnancy.
8. Fetal doses can classically remain within recommended limits without changes in occupational aims.
9. Staff remaining in the examination room must wear ear protectors during a scan.

- Anesthetist must ensure that regulations are appropriate.
- The effects of these hazards may be minimized by remaining in the control room while the scan is taking place.
- They must not be taken into the vicinity of the MRI scanner.
- Anesthetists, other staff and patients must be screened for the presence of any such implants.

- There is no evidence for an accumulative dangerous effect of strong magnetic fields, although temporary symptoms of may occur; safe levels of exposure are recommended.
- Monitoring by Health and Safety Executive.

Inhalational waste gases and the female anesthesiologist

Causes of inhalational waste gases operating room contamination:

- Inhalation induction.
- Mask ventilation.
- Leaks around uncuffed pediatric tracheal tubes.
- Unchanged of theatre air.
- Gas scavenging.

Effects of inhalational anesthetics waste gas on female anesthetics:

- Hepatic disease.
- Reduced mental concentration.
- Decreased manual handiness.
- Higher rate of spontaneous abortion .
- Increased incidence of congenital abnormalities in children of both male and female.

Diathermy and laser smoke inhalation:

- The median diameter of particles produced in smoke plumes is 0.31 μm.Surgical masks do not prevent toxic gases particles <0.5 μm in diameter.
- Inhalation of smoke from tissues treated with a carbon dioxide laser, and the smoke cloud generated by diathermy may contains:
1. Carcinogens such as benzene.

2. Chemicals (e.g. toluene, styrene, carbon disulphide corneal irritation, dermatitis, renal and hepatic toxicity and affect the central nervous system.

3. bacteria, human papillomavirus DNA and HIV proviral DNA

Operator exposure can be reduced effectively by suction devices.

Electromagnetic fields ,and female anesthesiologist:

- Increased risk of brain cancer,
- Breast cancer
- leukemia
- Female anesthetists should minimize their exposure.

Musculoskeletal injuries:

Wounds and glass splinters when opening drug ampoules are a common occurrence.

Plastic ampoules or ,plastic 'ampoule snappers' should be used.

The first metacarpo-phalyngeal joint osteoarthritis causes:

- Hand ventilation,
- Opening ampoules.
- Drawing up injecting drugs.

Repetitive strain injury

Holding of facemasks for prolonged periods is increasingly rare after the introduction of the laryngeal mask airway.

Lower lemb muscle sprain may occur due to prolonged standing.

Varicose vein

Latex allergy:

Due to repeated latex exposure.:it may cause

- Irritant contact dermatitis.
- A delayed type IV reaction mediated by T-cells to IgE-mediated anaphylactic shock.

Protection against latex allergy:
- The use of latex free products
- Hand washing after contact with latex containing products
- Educational programmes to reduce the prevalence of latex allergy.
- Atopic anesthesiologist should take latex allergy in considerations.

Addiction and anesthesiologist:

- Female anesthesiologists are less drug abuser than male.
- Below 40 yr are more than older.
- Anesthesiologists with Socioeconomic problems are more than others.

The most of drugs abused are:

- Opioids, benzodiazepines
- Dependence on highly lipid soluble opioids such as fentanyl develops rapidly and an affected individual requires ever increasing doses of the drug as tolerance develops.

Specific risk factors for anesthesiology addiction:

1. Genetic predisposition may precipitate the development of chemical dependence.
2. Anesthetists give drugs directly to the patient rather than prescribing them for others to administer. This
3. ready access to a wide range of potent psychoactive drugs
4. a detailed knowledge of pharmacology.
5. Anesthetists usually work alone and may feel they have less control over their professional lives than colleagues in other specialties.
6. The threat of medico legal proceedings can be an enormous burden.
7. Consideration of non-professional pressures (e.g. financial, marital) must also be given in the understanding of drug abuse and dependence.

Signs and symptoms of drug out side hospital :

Neglect and deterioration in appearance

Mood swings (e.g. depression, anger, irritability, paranoia, elation)

Fatigue and lethargy

Poor concentration, memory, confusion and impaired judgement

Frequent unexplained illness

Domestic instability

Legal problems (e.g. driving while under the influence of drink, drugs, or both)

Financial difficulties, gambling and fraud

Frequent house moves or job changes

Drugs and alcohol found at home, offices or inappropriate places (e.g. car)

Smell of alcohol on breath

Weight loss

Table 3

Signs and symptoms of chemical dependence seen in the hospital

Difficult relationships with colleagues

Mood swings (e.g. depression, anger, irritability, paranoia, elation)

Unreliable, poor time keeping

Poor administration and record keeping

Disproportionate levels of postoperative pain in patients when compared with apparently administered drugs

Progressive increase in use of narcotics and other drugs for anaesthetic management

Inconsistencies in recording and unaccountable missing drugs

Preference for working alone

Frequent requests to use the toilet

Difficult to find between cases or when on call

Often appears at the hospital when not on call

Unusual willingness to take on extra work commitments

Carrying syringes and ampoules in clothing

Bloody swabs and syringes in inappropriate places (e.g. offices)

Wearing of long sleeved gowns (to hide track marks and prevent chills seen in early withdrawal)

Pinpoint pupils when using or dilated pupils when withdrawing (opioids)

Smell of alcohol on breath

Found comatose or dead

Witnessed self-administration

Oxford JournalsMedicine & HealthBJA: CEACCPVolume 6, Issue 5Pp. 182-187

Management of drug addicted anesthesiologists:

1. Education of all personnel should allow early identification and treatment of anesthetists with a drug
2. appropriate treatment can be instigated before serious consequences have occurred, either for the individual or their patients.
3. Colleagues may also choose to believe implausible excuses offered by an individual rather than see a friend and colleague labelled as a 'drug addict'.
4. Accessible protocols allowing confidential reporting of suspected or actual drug abuse, alcohol abuse, or both must be followed.

Returning to work after treatement:

- Change the place workplace if it was contributory factor in the original problem
- Random testing used to monitor abstinence.

Factors increase the risk of relapse includes:

- addiction to an opioid,
- coexisting psychiatric illness,

- A family history of substance misuse
- A history of previous relapse.

Mortality:

- Mortality risk attributable to suicide,
- Deaths related to drugs,
- HIV.
- Cerebrovascular disease.

High mortality risk anesthesiologists:

- Mental illness,
- Personal difficulties,
- Occupational work stress,
- Substance abuse
- Access to material in order to accomplish suicide.

Stress:

- Mental and physical stress.
- Moderate levels of stress are an important driving factor in optimizing performance.

predisposing factors increasing feeling with sress:

- Individual personality type is a significant factor in the development of stress.
- Coping mechanisms of the same work.
- Mental illness,
- Familial, marital and financial problems.
- Occupational work stress.
- Medico legal problems.
- Substance abuse

Effect of stressed anesthesiologist on performance their jobs:

- Decreased job satisfaction.
- Impairment of decision making.
- Suicide.
- Chronic exposure to stress will lead to exhaustion, characterized by physical and emotional symptoms, mental dysfunction and,

    Management of stress and decrease its effects:
    - Recognition of its nature and causes.
    - Modifications to lifestyle can then be made before clinical skills become impaired.

Stress and female fertility life:

- Continuous stress mediates stress-induced inhibition of reproductive
- The anatomical sites at which these effects take place affected with sress.
- The role of hormones or neurotransmitters released during stress.
- At the level of the gonads, adrenal corticoids, pro-opiomelanocortin (POMC)-like peptides, and corticotropin-releasing factor (CRF) are

reported to interfere with the stimulatory action of gonadotropins on sex steroid-producing cells.

- Increased circulating corticosteroid levels may also decrease pituitary responsiveness to GnRH.
- that these mechanisms are primarily involved in mediating the effects of prolonged stress, but not those of an acute stimulus
- Hormones or neurotransmitters, including CRF, POMC peptides, and biogenic amines act within the brain to mediate the inhibitory influence of both acute and prolonged stresses on reproductive function.

Psychosocial factors and pregnancy outcome:

1. birth weight,
2. preeclampsia,
3. preterm labour
4. spontaneous abortion
5. Malformed or growth-retarded .
6. intrapartum complications.

There are three mechanisms for preterm labour with continuous stress:

(1) An indirect effect of unhealthy coping and life style behavior,

(2) a direct effect of stress-dependent hormones,

(3) an additional direct influence via psycho-immunological factors.

Fatigue

1. **Sleep loss and disruption of circadian rhythm**
- Reduced attention and vigilance,
- Poor memory,
- Impaired decision making,
- Prolonged reaction time
- Disrupted communications.
- Fatigue-related incidents a result of the individual 'microsleeps'(uncontrolled and spontaneous episodes of physiological sleep may last seconds or minutes).
- Reduce performance sufficiently which is against safety risks.
2. Workload pressures,
3. Insufficient numbers of personnel.
4. Hypovolemia, hypoglycemia, alcohol and drug use, poor general health and concomitant use of some prescription medications.
5. Increasing complexity of procedures compound.

Chronic fatigue on individual's physical health:

- Peptic ulcer disease.
- Non-specific abdominal symptoms.
- The incidence of cardiovascular disorders.

Effects of evening and night shifts, rotating or changing schedules, and the irregularity of work patterns on to reproductive outcome :

- Nonstandard work hours may disturb normal body functions
- Newly published studies suggest an association between rotating shift work and prolonged waiting time to pregnancy.
- Spontaneous abortion suggests that some forms of shift work may be associated with increased risk.
- Previous studies indicate that shift work including night schedules may be related to preterm birth.
- Moreover, some results have related rotating schedules to intrauterine growth retardation. This is unclear, to consider shift work as a potential risk to reproduction , but must take care of this piont.

Physical Work Load and pregnancy:

Continuous physical exertion effects on important determinants of embryonic and fetal development and survival:

1. intraabdominal pressure
2. uterine blood flow
3. hormonal balance
4. Nutritional status.

Effects of fatigue on Pregnancy Outcome:

- gestational age/premature birth,
- Birth weight/intrauterine growth retardation,
- Spontaneous abortion.
- Exhausting work, especially when involving long hours of standing and walking, seems to increase the risk of preterm delivery.
- The effect on intrauterine growth and spontaneous abortion risk is less clear.
- Heavy lifting has in most circumstances not been associated with a significantly increased risk of these outcomes.
- Enough rest periods assured, especially in late pregnancy.

Strategies to reduce fatigue-related incidents include

- Relief planning,
- Regular and

- Rehearsed equipment checking routines,
- Improved workplace design (including drug ampoule and syringe labelling protocols).
- Regulation of working hours.
- Regulate feeding time to prevent hypoglycemia and hypovolemia.
- Decrease caffeine intake.

<u>Plans to maintain alertness:</u>
- Nap wherever possible for 45 min or >2 h
- Overcome sleep inertia by increasing light levels, stretching, walking briskly and taking refreshment
- Alert colleagues if microsleeps/nodding off occurs and ask for relief
- Whenever relief is available, take a break
- Caffeinated drinks
- If working next day, nap rather than working through
- Nap before driving home
- Post call, sleep rather than party to pay off sleep debt. Go to bed earlier than normal

Female anesthesiologist and family:

The beneficial effects of working mothers and her family

- Support the finance of the family ,enhance better housing, children education , and health care.
- Women can share in the development of economy and her country welfare.
- Women may be talented in some specialty may be as scientist, and hving many ideas, and may be a figure in her community.
- Satisfaction in her work, and high level of education improve her knowledge about her children care, working mothers are more sensitive to her children.
- Mothers-children relationship and the mothesr need for continous financial support may increase success in her work.

The draw backs of high education and work of women:

- Delayed marriage and motherhood. The new home economy play an important role in women decision for marriage and mother hood.
- **Parents' working hours were driven by the requirements**
  Jobs, income, and the cultures of their workplaces, as well as the satisfaction work provided may affect emotional status of working mothers.
- Failure of working women to reduce their hours, had negative impacts on family life.
- **factors mediated the impact of long hours of work,**

1. The availability of extended family for childcare and support.
2. Having flexible work arrangements
3. control over hours of work
4. How satisfied options were with both the number of hours of paid work and the impact of these hours on the availability of the long-hours worker to spend time with children.
5. Father help in supporting working mothers ,and increases family stability.

Factors affecting working mother in caring her children:
1. **Marital status and family structure**: working mothers who are married to the fathers of their children have more stable families
2. **Type of work**: Working mothers in business or the professions usually receive more than women with less education and often find their work psychologically satisfying. The night shifts, and the disturbed schedule ,or emergency call may make ,distraction , psychological stress, anxiety, with dealing with her children.
3. **Income level**: Working mothers with well-paying jobs have more choices about housing, transportation, and child care arrangements than those with limited incomes.
4. **Number, ages, and special needs of children:**
    i. equal,
    ii. women with fewer,
    iii. widely spaced
    iv. Healthy children find it easier to juggle than whose children suffer from chronic illnesses or developmental difficulties.

5. **Age of working mothers** :

- Mothers over 40 are more likely to develop job-related health problems than younger women.
- Women in this age group are often coping with the care of aging parents as well as their own offspring.

Role of working mothers in the different children age groups:

Infants age groups

Maternity leave Payment leave time usually very small to satisfy infant need.

During infant age the female anesthesiologist usually during residanancy and training stage. Night shifts, emergency schedule may interfere with regular breast feeding:

Common problems facing infants of female anesthestis:

- Respiratory illness is far more common among formula-fed children. Infants are at greater risk of being hospitalized with a severe respiratory infection than do infants breast-fed for a minimum of four months.

- Diarrheal disease is three to four times more likely to occur in infants fed formula than those fed breast milk.

- Breastfeeding has been shown to reduce the likelihood of ear infections, and to prevent recurrent ear infections.

- In developing countries, differences in infection rates can seriously affect an infant's chances for survival..

- Researchers have observed a decrease in the probability of Sudden Infant Death Syndrome (SIDS) in breast-fed infants.

- Another apparent benefit from breastfeeding may be protection from allergies. Eczema, an allergic reaction, is significantly rarer in breast-fed babies.

Benefits to the Child Later in Life:

Some benefits of breastfeeding on older child .

- Infants who are breast-fed longer have fewer dental cavities throughout their lives.
- Less likely to become obese later in childhood.

- Children who are exclusively breast-fed during the first three months of their lives are 34 percent less likely to develop juvenile, insulin-dependent diabetes than children who are fed formula.

- Decrease the risk of childhood cancer in children less than 15 years of age.

- Breast-fed as infants have lower blood pressure on average than those who were formula-fed.

- Significant evidence suggests that breast-fed children develop fewer psychological, behavioral and learning problems as they grow older.

- Psychological benefits of breast milk, breast-fed children were, on average, more mature, assertive and secure with themselves as they developed.

Benefits to the Mother:

- A woman grows both physically and emotionally from the relationship she forms with her baby.
- Breastfeeding helps a woman to lose weight after birth.
- Breastfeeding releases a hormone in the mother (oxytocin) that causes the uterus to return to its normal size more quickly.
- When a woman gives birth and proceeds to nurse her baby, she protects herself from becoming pregnant again too soon,
- Breastfeeding appears to reduce the mother's risk of developing osteoporosis in later years. Although mothers experience bone-mineral loss during breastfeeding, their mineral density is replenished and even increased after lactation.
- Diabetic women improve their health by breastfeeding and decreases the amount of insulin that the mother requires postpartum period.
- Women who lactate for a total of two or more years reduce their chances of developing breast cancer by 24 percent.
- Women who breastfeed their children have been shown to be less likely to develop uterine, endometrial or ovarian cancer.
- The emotional health of the mother may be enhanced by the relationship she develops with her infant during breastfeeding, resulting in fewer feelings of anxiety and a stronger sense of connection with her baby.

- A woman's ability to produce all of the nutrients that her child needs can provide her with a sense of confidence. Researchers have pointed out that the bond of a nursing mother and child is stronger than any other human contact.

Social and Economic Benefits of Breastfeeding:

- Women who breastfeed avoid the financial burden of buying infant formula, an average expense of $800 per year.

Breast-fed babies are less likely to need excessive medical attention as they grow.

Health problems facing the children of female anesthestis

- Asthma episode within the past 12 months,
- injury or poisoning
- Less time to prepare healthy meals or clean the home.
- Timing of regular vaccination, and medical consolation.

The Impact of Working Mothers on Child Development:

- Work stress and depression may affect their Infants to have difficulties with self-quieting, lower activity levels and decreased ability to attend.
- Be hyper-vigilant with their child.
- focus on the negative, while ignoring improved behavior;
- engage in coercive and punitive parenting;

- misread neutral child cues as malevolent,
- Derogate child in efforts at power repair.
- High levels of resistance, and at-risk behavior in the adolescent.
- A critical period in terms of attachment and emotional and cognitive growth is more likely to be associated with subsequent difficulties.
- Full-time working mothers started before the child was three months old was associated with significantly more behavior .
- Children whose mothers worked part-time before their child was one year old had fewer disruptive behavioral problems than the children of mothers who worked full-time before their child's first birthday. This increased risk for behavioral difficulties was apparent at age three, and during first grade.

- The pathway through which those protective effects of part-time work operated was through increases in the quality of the home environment and in the mother's sensitivity.
- Children of mothers who worked full-time in the first year of that child's life received modestly lower child cognitive scores relative to children of mothers who do not work on all eight cognitive outcomes examined. Associations at 4½ years and first grade were roughly similar in size to those at age three;
- Mothers who worked full-time were more likely to have symptoms of depression.
- Higher levels of maternal sensitivity seen in employed mothers might have stemmed from their having greater financial security.

- Children of working mothers showed higher levels of achievement and lower levels of internalizing behaviors such as anxiety and depression.

<u>Female anesthetist and, her children in school</u>

Waking up kids

Placing out each their school uniform,

Preparing breakfast for them and to make sure that each one is done with his breakfast,

Make school lunch boxes

Dressing them up in uniform

Checking their bags and sending them school timely.

Mother has to be capable of solving daily emerging puzzles and problems.

She performs simultaneously including maternal role, spousal role and community role.

Follow-up of performing homework and academic level Raising children on Moral, to respect the general laws, and provide assistance to those in need.

<u>Family stress on female anesthetist may affect her work</u>:

1. Feeling guilt that she is not herself able to look after her kids all the time
2. Worrying about that she is not able to do her work with due concentration which she was supposed to do.
3. Persistent feeling of guilt leading to stress and costing her health.
4. Sleep well or not during night due to health problem for her or for her kids.

Strategies to decrease the effect of the effect of working hours absence on the offspring:

- Regulation of work schedule, night shift must be suitable for caring of young children.

- Training residency may be prolonged for mother anesthetist to give her the chance for education, training, and caring of her children.

- Continuous monitoring of the general health and psychological support for female anesthetist.

- Continuous education of the recent marriage couples about children care.

- Governmental health care support can introduce qualified nursing centers.

- High-quality childcare for children.

- The father should make an effort to be present in as active a parenting role as possible.

- Grand parents should be more actively recruited to take care of their grandchildren when they are infants and both parents are working full-time.

Family gap:

Female anesthesiologist confronted by 2 types of family gaps:

I.   Family gap due to the difference in payment between women and men.

II.   Family gap between female anesthesiologist with, and without children

Family gap is the difference in payment between women and men

- It has been narrowed nowadays.
- Female anesthesiologists spent only 1.6 fewer hours per week in medical and administrative activities than male anesthesiologists did.
- Female physicians had smaller net incomes within each of the years-of-experience categories; and female physicians attained their highest earnings earlier than their male colleagues did.
- Several factors may explain the net income discrepancy.

1. A larger number of self-employed physicians are male,

2. Physician entrepreneurs receive greater rewards than their staff-employed colleagues do differences in the number of hours spent in medical and administrative activities and by differences in the number of patient visits per week.

3. Female physicians spent fewer hours in work-related activities and saw fewer patients each week.

4. Female anesthesiologist spent the same official schedule as the male coellegue,in night shift ,emergency schedule.

5. More hours for private work is difficult for female anesthesiologist with children, however she want to raise her income , she spent more time with her children.

6. In developing countries there is still sex discrimination based on traditional thinking as male and female are in equal ,so private work of female anesthesiologist may be less.

7. Female anesthesiologist with children may have limited time to take more upgrading courses as sonar guided block or ICU block which may be a factor in less income than male colleague.

I. **Family gap between female anesthesiologist with, and without children**

Causes of widening the gap between women with children and those without children :

1. The main motivation behind this reform 2 was the health of the mother; it was argued that the female body takes longer than two months to fully recover from pregnancy.

2. The main motivation behind these reforms was the welfare of the child; it was argued that the early years are the most important ones in a child's life.

3. Leave policies improve of the health of the mother and the welfare of the child, explicitly aimed at encouraging mothers to spend more time with their child after childbirth.

4. The institutional structure it has emphasized equal pay and equal opportunity policies, but not family policies such as maternity leave and child care.

5. Countries that have implemented family policies along with their gender policies seem to have had better success at narrowing both the gender gap and the family gap.

6. Although much of the evidence on links between family policies and women's pay is speculative, there is one policy maternity leave .Recent research in the United States, as well as comparative research on Britain and Japan, suggests that maternity leave coverage may raise.

7. Up to 7 % of women return to work exactly when leave expires, but become unemployed only one or two months later.

8. Every country has provisions for maternity leave allowing mothers to leave their workplace for a limited time around childbirth, and giving them the right to return to their previous employer afterwards. However, these provisions vary widely across countries.

9. However the widespread prevalence of parental leave policies, there is economic impact.

10. Encouraging employment continuity, parental leave policies promote gender equality and increase women's earnings.

11. Restricting voluntary agreements between firms and workers, leave policies worsen women's position in the labor market.

Author Recommendations:

Support female anesthesiologist especially in developing countries. Starting to narrow the family gap,

Maternity leave adjustment for:

6. Keeping skills and experience by extended courses of training for female anesthesiologist with children.

7. Financial support for female anesthesiologist, maintain children welfare as much as time spent with them.

8. The community and country development may use the double benefit from continuous support of working women, from her work, and from normal physical and emotional children.

9. Continuous medical super vision against hazards of infection and radiation ,with special attention during pregnancy.

10. Community support motivates working women to get achievement in both work and children.

Suggested readings and references:

1. Ahlborg, Gunnar Jr. MD Physical Work Load and Pregnancy Outcome.**Journal of Occupational & Environmental Medicine: Abstract**

2. (C)1995The American College of Occupational and Environmental Medicine

3. Makuc D: Employment characteristics of mothers during pregnancy. In: National Center for Health Statistics, PHS, DHHS: Health, United States, 176 AJPH February 1990, Vol. 80, No. 2 WORK STRESS AND PREGNANCY OUTCOME 1983. Hyattsville, MD, 1983;25-31.

4. Committee to Study the Prevention of Low Birthweight (Behrman R, chair): Preventing Low Birthweight. Washington, DC: National Academy Press, 1985;71-2

5. Stein ZA, Susser MW, Hatch MC: Working during pregnancy: physical and psychosocial strain. State Art Rev Occup Med 1986; 1:405-409.

6. Fox ME, Harris RE, Brekken AL: The active duty military pregnancy: A new high risk category. Am J Obstet Gynecol 1977; 129:705-707.

7. Mamelle N, Laumon B, Lazar P: Prematurity and occupational activity during pregnancy. Am J Epidemiol 1984; 119:30.

8. Joffe M: Biases in research on reproduction and women's work. Int J Epidemiol 1985; 14:118-123.

9. Kasl SV: Stress and Health. Annu Rev Public Health 1984; 5:319-341.

10. Karasek RA, Theorell TFT, Schwartz J, Schall PL, Pieper C, Michela JL: Job characteristics in relation to the prevalence of myocardial infarction in

the US Health Examination Survey and the Health and Nutrition Examination Survey. Am J Public Health 1988; 78:910-918.

11. Karasek RA, Baker D, Marxer F, Ahlbom A, Theorell R: Job decision latitude, job demands, and cardiovascular disease: a prospective study of Swedish men. Am J Public Health 1981; 71:694-705.

12. Wolpin K: The National Longitudinal Surveys handbook 1983-1984. Columbus, OH: Ohio State University, 1983.

13. Mott FL: Evaluation of Fertility Data and Preliminary Analytic Results for the 1983 (5th Round) Survey of the National Longitudinal Survey of Labor Market Experience, Youth Cohort. Columbus, OH: Ohio State University, 1985.

14. Schwartz JE, Pieper CF, Karasek RA: A procedure for linking psychosocial job characteristics data to health surveys. Am J Public Health 1988; 78:904-909. 13. Quinn RP, Staines GL: The 1977 Quality of Employment Surveys: descriptive statistics with comparison data for the 1969-70 and the 1972-73 surveys. Ann Arbor, MI: Institute for Social Research, 1979.

15. Harrell FE, Jr: The LOGIST procedure. In: SAS Institute, Inc: SUGI Supplemental Library User's Guide. Cary, NC: SAS Institute, 1985.

16. Frankel MR, McMullen HA, and Spencer B: National Longitudinal Survey of Labor Force Behavior Youth Survey, Technical Sampling Report. Chicago, IL: National Opinion Research Center, 1983.

17. LaCroix AZ: Occupational Exposure to high demand/low control work and coronary heart disease incidence in the Framingham cohort. PhD Dissertation, University of North Carolina at Chapel Hill, 1984.

18. Karasek RA, Theorell TFT, Schwartz J, Pieper C, Alfredson L: Job, psychological factors, and coronary heart disease. Adv Cardiol 1982; 29:62-67.

19. National Center for Health Statistics, Pamuk ER, Mosher WD: Health aspects of pregnancy and childbirth, US, 1982. Vital and health statistics Series 23, No. 16, DHHS Pub No (PHS) 89-1992 PHS. Washington, DC: Govt Printing Office, 1989.

20. Kleinbaum D, Kupper L, Morgenstern H: Epidemiologic Research: Principles and Quantitative Methods. Belmont, CA: Lifetime Learning Publications, 1982.

21. National Center for Health Statistics, Taffel S: Matemal weight gain and the outcome of pregnancy, US, 1980. Vital and health statistics Series 21, No. 44, DHHS Pub No (PHS) 86-1922. Washington, DC: Govt Printing Office, 1986.

22. Frieden TR, Sterling TR, Munsiff SS, Walt CJ, Dye C. Tuberculosis. Lancet 2003;362:887-99

23. Global Tuberculosis Control: Surveillance, planning, financing: WHO report. Geneva: World Health Organization; 2007

24. Trends in tuberculosis - United States 2007. MMWR Morb Mortal wkly Rep 2008;57:281-5.

25. Schaefer G. Female genital tuberculosis. Clin Obstet Gynecol 1976;19:223-39.

26. Muir DG, Belsey MA. Pelvic inflammatory disease and its consequences in the developing world. Am J Obstet Gynecol 1980;138:913-28

27. Focus on Tuberculosis: Annual surveillance report 2006 - England, Wales and Northern Ireland. London: Health Protection Agency Centre for infection; 2006.

28. Corbett EL, Walt CJ, Walker N, Maher D, Williams BG, Raviglione MC, *et al*. The growing burden of tuberculosis; Global trends and interaction with HIV epidemic. Arch Intern Med 2003;163:1009-21

29. Arora VK, Gupta R, Arora R. Female genital tuberculosis - need for more research. Indian J Tuberc 2003;50:9-11

30. Choudhary NN. Overview of tuberculosis of the finance genital tract. J Med Assoc 1996;94:345-61.

31. Zignol M, Hosseini MS, Wright A, Weezenbeek CL, Nunn P, Watt CJ, *et al.* Global Incidence of multi drug resistant tuberculosis J Infect Dis 2006;194:479-95.

32. Shah NS, Wright A, Bai GH, Barrera L, Boulahbal F, Martín-Casabona N, *et al.* Worldwide emergence of exclusively drug resistant tuberculosis. Emerg Infect Dis 2007:13:380-7

33. Behera D. Tuberculosis control in India - a view point India. J Tuberc 2007;54:63-5.

34. Gopi PG, Subramani R, Santha T, Chandrashekhar V, Kolappan C, Selva Kumar N, *et al.* Estimation of the burden of tuberculosis in India for the year 2000. IJMR 2005;122:243-8.

35. Singh MM, XDR - TB - Danger ahead. Indian J Tuberc 2007:54:1-2

36. Roy H, Roy S. Use of polymerase chain reaction for the diagnosis of endometrial tuberculosis in high risk infertile women in an epidemic zone. J Obstet Gynaecol India 2003;53:260-3

37. Fallahian M, Tikhani M. Menstrual disorder in nongenital tuberculosis. Infect Dis Obstet Gynaecol 2006;18452:1-3

38. Sharma S. Menstrual dysfunction in non genital tuberculosis. Int J Gynaecol Obstet 2002;79:223-9.

39. Tripathy SN. Hormone profile of female cases of pulmonary tuberculosis. Indian J Tuberc 1994:41:223-8.

40. Kumar A, Rattan A. Anti gonadotrophic effect of *mycobacterium tuberculosis.* Horm Metabol 1997;29:501-6.

41. Tripathy SN. Genital manifestation of pulmonary tuberculosis. Int J Gynaecol Obstet 1981;19:319-26.

42. Arora VK, Bedi RS, Arora R. Rifampicin induced menstrual disturbances. Indian J Chest Dis Allied Sci 1987;29:63-7.

43. Keita N, Koulibaly M, Hijazy Y, Diallo M, Diop D, Diallo S, *et al*. Aspects of genital tuberculosis in women. Contracept Fertil Sex 1999;27:155-61.

44. Dawn CS. Pelvic Inflammation in Dawn CS. Ed. Text book of Gynecology and Contraception; 9 th ed. 1998. p 321. Arati Dawn Kolkata, India

45. Crofton J, Horne N, Miller F. Clinical tuberculosis. 1 st ed. London: Macmillan; 1992. p. 502-10.

46. Klein TA, Richmond JA, Mishell DR. Pelvic tuberculosis. Obstet Gynecol 1976;48:99-104.

47. Samal S, Gupta U, Agarwal P. Menstrual disorder in genital tuberculosis. J Indian Med Assoc 2000;98:126-9

48. Good JT, Iseman MD, Davidson PT, Lakshminarayan S, Sahn SA. Tuberculosis in association with pregnancy. Am J Obstet Gynecol 1981;140:492-8.

49. Demarch AP. Tuberculosis and Pregnancy five to 10 years review of 215 patients in their fertile age. Chest 1975;68:800-

50. Hamadeh MA, Glassroth J. Tuberculosis and pregnancy. Chest 1992;101:1114-20.

51. Wilson EA, Thelin TJ, Dilts PV. Tuberculosis complicated by pregnancy. Am J Obstet Gynecol 1973;115;526-7.

52. World Health Organization. World Health report 1999. 12368.

53. Kothari A, Mahadewan N, Girling J. Tuberculosis in pregnancy - Result of a study in high prevalence area in London. Eur J Obstet Gynecol Reprod Biol 2006;126:48-55.

54. LLewyn M, Gropley I, Wilkinson RJ, Davidson RN. Tuberculosis diagnosed during pregnancy: A prospective study from London. Thorax 2000;55 :129-32.

55. Figneroa-Ddomain R, Arredondo-Garcia JL. Neonatal outcome of children born to women with tuberculosis. Med Res 2001;2:66-99.

56. Tripathy SN. Tuberculosis and pregnancy. Int J Gynaecol Obstet 2003;80:247-53.

57. Carter EJ, Mates S. Tuberculosis during pregnancy. The Rhode Iseland experience, 1987 to 1991. Chest 1994;106:1466-70.

58. Lichtenstein MR. Tuberculosis reaction in pregnancy. Am Rev Respir Dis 1975;112:413-6.

59. Present PA, Cornstock GW. Tuberculosis sensitivity in pregnancy. Am Rev

Respir Dis 1975;112:413-6.

60. Bjerkedal TR, Bahna SL, Lehman EH. Course and outcome of pregnancy in women with pulmonary tuberculosis. Scand J Respir Dis 1975;56:245-50.

61. Jana N, Vashista K, Jindal S, Khuller B, Ghosh K. Perinatal out come in pregnancies complicated by pulmonary tuberculosis. Int J Gynaecol Obstet 1994;44:119-24.

62. Jana N, Vashista K, Saha SC, Ghosh K. Obstetrical outcome among women with extra pulmonary tuberculosis. N Engl J Med 1999;341:645-9.

63. Heywood S, Amoa AB, Mola GL, Klufio CA. A survey of pregnant women with tuberculosis at the post Moves by General Hospital. PNG Med J 1999;42:63-70

64. Snider D. Pregnancy and Tuberculosis Cohort. Chest 1984;86:105-35.

65. Ormerod P. Tuberculosis in pregnancy and puerperium. Thorax 2000;56:494-9.

66. Schaefer G, Zervoudakis IA, Fuchs FF, David S. Pregnancy and pulmonary tuberculosis. Obstet Gynaecol 1975;46:706-15.

67. Singh H, Singh J, Abdullah BT, Mathews A. Tuberculosis paraplegia in pregnancy treated by surgery. Singapore. Med J 2002;43:251-3.

68. Govender S, Moodly SC, Grootboom MJ. Tuberculosis paraplegia during pregnancy: A report of four cases. S Afr Med J 1989;75:190-2.

69. Kingdom JC, Kennedy DH. Tuberculosis meningitis in pregnancy. Br J Obstet Gynaecol 1989;96:233-5.

70. Arora VK, Gupta R. Tuberculosis and pregnancy. Indian J Tuberc 2003;50:13-6.

71. Stark JR. Tuberculosis. An old disease but a new threat to mother, fetus and neonate. Clin Perinatol 1997;24:107-14.

72. Cantwell MF, Shehab ZM, Costello AM, Sands L, Green WF, Ewing EP Jr, *et al.* Brief report: Congenital tuberculosis. N Engl J Med 1994;330:1051-3.

73. Franks AL, Binkin NJ, Snider DE Jr, Rowak WM, Becker S. Isoniazid hepatitis among pregnant and post partum Hispanic patients. Public Health Rep 1989; 104:151-5

74. Katoch VM. Newer diagnostic techniques for tuberculosis. Indian J Med Res 2004;120:418-28.

75. Alexander, M. and J. Baxter (2005) "Impacts of work on family life among partnered parents of young children" Family Matters, 72: 18--25.

76. Baxter, J. (2007) "When Dad works long hours: how work hours are associated with fathering 4--5-year-old children" Family Matters, 77:60--69.

77. Behnke, A. and S. MacDermid (2004) Family Wellbeing:SloanWork--FamilyNetwork,http://wfnetwork.bc.edu/encyclopedia_entry.php?id=235&area=All [accessed 12 March 2008].

78. Bianchi, S.M., J. Robinson and M. Milkie (2006) Changing Rhythms of American Family Life, Russell Sage Foundation, New York, NY.

79. Callister, P. (2004) Changes in Working Hours for Couples, 1985 to 2001. Labour, Employment and Work in New Zealand Conference, 22–23 November 2004,

80. WellingtoCrouter, A., M.F. Bumpus, M.R. Head and S. McHale (2001) "Implications of overwork and overload for the quality of men's family

relationships" Journal of Marriage and Family, 63(May):404--416.

81. Crouter, A., M. Bumpus, M. Maguire and S. McHale (1999) "Linking parents' work pressure and adolescents' wellbeing: insights into dynamics in dual-earner families" Developmental Psychology, 35:1453--1461.

82. Brost BC, Newman RB. The maternal and fetal effects of tuberculosis therapy. Obstet Gynecol Clin North Am 1997;24:659-73.

83. Crouter, A., K. Davis, K. Updegraff, M. Delgado and M. Fortner (2006) "Mexican American fathers' occupational conditions: links to family members' psychological adjustment" Journal of Marriage and Family,68: 843--858.

84. Department of Labour (2006) Work-life Balance in New Zealand: A Snapshot of Employee and Employer Attitudes and Experiences, Department of Labour, Wellington.

85. Department of Trade and Industry (2007) The Third Work-life Balance Employee Survey: Main Findings, Employment Relations Research Series No. 58

86. Dermott, E. (2006) "What's parenthood got to do with it?": men's hours of paid work" British Journal of Sociology, 57(4):619--634.

87. Families Commission (2008) Give and Take: Families' Perceptions and Experiences of Flexible Work in New Zealand, Families Commission, Wellington.

88. Fursman, L. (2008) Working Long Hours in New Zealand: A Profile of Long Hours Workers Using Data from the 2006 Census, Department of Labour and the Families Commission, Wellington.

89. Galambos, N., H. Sears, D. Almeida and G. Kolaric (1995) "Parents' work overload and problem behaviour in young adolescents" Journal of Research

on Adolescence, 5:201--223.

90. Hird, S. (2003) Individual Wellbeing: A Report for the Scottish Executive and Scottish Neighbourhood Statistics [accessed 12 March 2008].

91. Maume, D.J. and M.L. Bellas (2001) "The overworked American or the time bind? assessing competing explanations for time spend in paid labor" American Behavioural Scientist, 44(7):1137--1156.

92. Messenger, J.C. (2004) "Finding the balance: working time and workers' needs and preferences in industrialized countries -- A summary of the report and its implications for working time policies" paper presented at the 9th International Symposium on Working Time, Paris, 26--28 February

93. Milligan, S., A. Fabian, P. Coope and C. Errington (2006) Family Wellbeing Indicators from the 1981--2001 New Zealand Censuses, Statistics New Zealand, University of Auckland and University of Otago [accessed 12 March 2008].

94. Ministry of Social Development (2006) Work, Family, and Parenting Study: Research Findings Relationships Forum (2007) An Unexpected Tragedy: Evidence for the Connection between Working Patterns and Family Breakdown in Australia

95. Strazdins, L., R.J. Korda, L. Lim, D.H. Broom and R. D'Souza (2004) "Around-the-clock: parent work schedules and children's wellbeing in a 24-h economy" Social Science and Medicine, 59:1517--1527.

96. Weston, R., M. Gray, L. Qu and D. Stanton (2004) Long Work Hours and the Wellbeing of Fathers and Their Families, Research Paper No. 35, Australian Institute of Family Studies, Melbourne.

97. Weston, R., L. Qu and G. Soriano (2002) "Implications of men's extended work hours for their personal and marital happiness" Family Matters, 61:18-

-25.

98. Hepatitis C; NICE CKS, March 2010 (UK access only)

99. Management of the viral hepatitides A, B and C; British Association for Sexual Health and HIV (2008)

100. Hepatitis C: guidance, data and analysis; Public Health England, April 2013

101. Nash KL, Bentley I, Hirschfield GM; Managing hepatitis C virus infection. BMJ. 2009 Jun 26;338:b2366. doi: 10.1136/bmj.b2366.

102. Management of co-infection with HIV-1 and hepatitis B or C virus; British HIV Association (2010)

103. British National Formulary; 69th Edition (Mar 2015) British Medical Association and Royal Pharmaceutical Society of Great Britain, London

104. Peginterferon alfa and ribavirin for the treatment of chronic hepatitis C; NICE Technology Appraisal Guideline, September 2010

105. Boceprevir for the treatment of genotype 1 chronic hepatitis C; NICE Technology Appraisal Guideline, April 2012

106. Telaprevir for the treatment of genotype 1 chronic hepatitis C; NICE Technology Appraisal Guideline, April 2012

107. Rowe IA, Mutimer DJ; Protease inhibitors for treatment of genotype 1 hepatitis C virus infection. BMJ. 2011 Nov 10;343:d6972. doi: 10.1136/bmj.d6972.

108. Wilby KJ, Partovi N, Ford JA, et al; Review of boceprevir and telaprevir for the treatment of chronic hepatitis C. Can J Gastroenterol. 2012 Apr;26(4):205-10.

109. Sofosbuvir for treating chronic hepatitis C; NICE Technology Appraisal Guideline, February 2015

110.   Simeprevir in combination with peginterferon alfa and ribavirin for treating genotypes 1 and 4 chronic hepatitis C; NICE Technology Appraisal Guideline, February 2015

111.   Peginterferon alfa and ribavirin for treating chronic hepatitis C in children and young people; NICE Technology Appraisal Guideline, November 2013

112.   Management of hepatitis C; Scottish Intercollegiate Guidelines Network - SIGN (July 2013)

113.   Ploss A, Dubuisson J; New advances in the molecular biology of hepatitis C virus infection: towards the Gut. 2012 May;61 Suppl 1:i25-35.

114.   Baumert TF, Fauvelle C, Chen DY, et al; A prophylactic hepatitis C virus vaccine: a distant peak still worth climbing. J Hepatol. 2014 Nov;61(1 Suppl):S34-44. doi: 10.1016/j.jhep.2014.09.009. Epub 2014 Nov 3.

115.   Askrog V, Harvald B. Teratogen effekt af inhalationsanestetika. Nord med 83 (1970) 498-500.

116.   Axelson 0, Andersson K, Hogstedt C, Holmberg B, Molina G, De Verdier A. A cohort study on trichloroethylene exposure and cancer mortality. J occup med 20 (1978) 194-196. 3.

117.   Baden JM, Brinckenhoff M, Wharton RS, Hitt BA, Simmon VF, Mazze R. Mutagenicity of volatile anesthetics: Halothane. Anesthesiology 45 (1976) 311-318.

118.   Baden JM, Kelley M, Wharton RF, Hitt B, Simmon VF, Mazze R. Mutagenicity of halogenated ether anesthetics. Anesthesiology 46 (1977) 346-350.

119.   Baltzar B, Ericson A, Kallen B. Delivery outcome in women employed in medical occupations in Sweden. J occup med 21 (1979) 543-

548.

120.   Belfrage S, Ahlgren J, Axelson S. Halothane hepatitis in an anesthetist. Lancet 2 (1966) 1466-1467. 7. Boyland E. Biochemistry of occupational cancer. J soc occup med 27 (1977) 97-101

121.   Bruce DL, Bach MJ. Trace effects of anesthetic gases on behavioral performance of operating room personnel. US Department of Health, Education and Welfare, Public Health Service, Center for Disease Control, National Institute for Occupational Safety and Health, Cincinnati, OH 1976. (HEW publication no (NIOSH) 76-169).

122.   Bruce DL, Eide KA, Linde HW, Eckenhoff JE. Causes of death among anesthesiologists - A 20-year survey. Anesthesiology 29 (1968) 565-569.

123.   Bruce DL, Eide KA, Smith MJ, Seltzer F, Dykes MHM. A prospective survey of anesthesiologists mortality 1967-1971. Anesthesiology 41 (1974) 71-74.

124.   Chang L, Dudley AW Jr, Katz J, Martin AH. Nervous system development following in utero exposure to trace amounts of halothane. Teratology 9 (1974) A-15.

125.   Chang LW, Dudley AW Jr, Lee YK, Katz J. Ultrastructural changes in the nervous system after chronic exposure to halothane. Exp neurol 45 (1974) 209-219.

126.   Chang LW, Dudley AW Jr, Lee YK, Katz J. Ultrastructural changes in the kidney following chronic exposure to low levels of halothane. Am j pathol 78 (1975) 225- 232.

127.   . Coate WB, Ulland BM, Lewis TR. Chronic exposure to low concentrations of halothane, nitrous oxide: Lack of carcinogenic effect in the

rat. Anesthesiology 50 (1979) 306-309.

128.   Cohen EN. Toxicity of inhalation anaesthetic agents. Br j anaesth 50 (1978) 665- 675. 16. Cohen EN, Brown BW, Bruce DL, Cascorbi HF, Corbett TH, Jones TW, Whitcher CH. Occupation disease among operating room personnel: A national study. Anesthesiology 41 (1974) 321-340.

129.   Ahmed Arif, Shaheed Zulfiqar Ali Bhutto: Impact of Long Working Hours on Family Wellbeing of Corporate Family ,World Applied Sciences Journal 16 (9): 1302-1307, 20.

130.   Schönberg, Uta; Ludsteck, Johannes Working Paper Maternity leave legislation, female labor supply, and the family wage gap IZA Discussion Papers, No. 2699 Provided in Cooperation with: Institute for the Study of Labor (IZA)

131.   B.H. Kehrer, "Factors Affecting the Incomes of Men and Women Physicians: An Explor- atory Analysis," Journal of Human Resources (Fall 1976): 526–545;

132.   K.M. Langwell, "Factors Affecting the Incomes of Men and Women Physicians: Further Explorations," Journal of Human Resources (Spring 1982): 261–274. 2. R.J.

133.   Ohsfeldt and S.D. Culler, "Differences in Income Between Male and Female Physi- cians," Journal of Health Economics (December 1984): 335–346. 3. Ibid.

134.   A B Silberger, W D Marder and R J Willke Practice characteristics of male and female physicians doi: 10.1377/hlthaff.6.4.104 Health Affairs, 6, no.4 (1987):104-109

135.

www.ingramcontent.com/pod-product-compliance
Lightning Source LLC
Chambersburg PA
CBHW070846180526
45168CB00002B/975